Contents

Anaphylaxis is a severe allergic reaction to venom, food, or medication. Most cases are caused by a bee sting or eating foods that are known to cause allergies, such as peanuts or tree nuts. Anaphylaxis causes a series of symptoms, including a rash, low pulse, and shock, which is known as anaphylactic shock.

ANAPHYLAXIS DIET RECIPES

BREAKFAST
1. Baked Eggs and Zoodles with Avocado
Ingredients

2 servings

- Nonstick spray
- 3 zucchini, spiralized into noodles
- 2 tablespoons extra-virgin oliveoil
- Kosher salt and freshly ground black pepper
- 4 largeeggs
- Red-pepper flakes, for garnishing
- Fresh basil, for garnishing
- 2 avocados, halved and thinly sliced

Direction

1. Preheat theoven to 350°F. Lightly greasea baking sheet with nonstick spray.
2. In a large bowl, toss the zucchini noodles and oliveoil to combine. Season with salt and pepper. Divide into 4 even portions, transfer to the baking sheet and shapeeach intoa nest.

3. Gently crack an egg into the center of each nest. Bake until theeggs are set, 9 to 11 minutes. Season with salt and pepper; garnish with red-pepper flakes and basil. Servealongside theavocado slices.

2. Banana MochaOvernight Oats

Prep Time: 10 Minutes

Total Time: 10 Minutes

Yields: 2 Servings

Ingredients

- 1 banana
- 3/4 cup almond milk or another non-dairy milk of choice
- 1/2 cup strong coffee cold brew works well
- 2 pitted dates if your blender isn't very strong, you can soak these in warm water for an hour, then drain before blending
- 2 tablespoons cocoa powder
- Pinch sea salt
- 1 cup rolled oats
- 1 1/2 tablespoons chia seeds
- Fresh fruit for serving

Instructions

1. Blend the banana, almond milk, coffee, dates, cocoa powder, and sea salt together in a blender till

smooth. Place theoats and chia seeds in an airtight container. Pour the liquid mixtureover theoats and chia seeds, then stir everything well to combine. Cover and refrigerateovernight.

2. In the morning, stir your oats again and add a small splash of additional non-dairy milk as needed. Top with fresh fruit and enjoy.

Ingredients

6 servings

- 8 eggs
- ⅓ cup milk
- 1 teaspoon dried oregano
- Salt and freshly ground black pepper, to taste
- 4 cups baby arugula
- 1¼ cups chopped roasted red peppers
- ½ cup thinly sliced red onion
- ¾ cup crumbled goat cheese

Directions

1. Grease the insideof the slow cooker with nonstick spray.

2. In a large bowl, whisk the eggs with the milk and oregano to combine. Season with salt and pepper to taste.

3. Arrange the baby arugula, roasted red peppers, red onion and goat cheese in the slow cooker. Pour theeggs over the vegetables.

4. Cook on low for 2½ to 3 hours. Serve immediately.

Ingredients

Breakfast Bowls Ingredients:

- 1 tablespoon avocadooil or oliveoil
- 1 pound asparagus[1], cut into bite-sized pieces *(with ends trimmed and discarded)*
- 3 cups shredded kale leaves
- 1 batch lemony dressing *(see recipe below)*
- 3 cups shredded (uncooked) Brussels sprouts[2]
- 1 ½ cups cooked quinoa[3]
- ½ cup hummus
- 1 avocado, peeled, pitted and thinly-sliced
- 4 eggs, cooked however you'd like *(I soft-boiled mine)*
- garnishes: sunflower seeds *(or sliced almonds)*, toasted sesame seeds, crushed red pepper

Lemony Dressing Ingredients:

- 2 tablespoons avocadooil or oliveoil

- 2 tablespoons freshly-squeezed lemon juice
- 2 teaspoons Dijon mustard
- 1 garlic clove, minced
- salt and freshly-cracked black pepper

Directions

To Make the Breakfast Bowls:

1. Heat oil in a large saute pan over medium-high heat. Add asparagus and saute for 4-5 minutes, stirring occasionally, until tender. Remove from heat and set side.
2. Meanwhile, in a large mixing bowl, combine the kaleand lemony dressing. Then use your fingers to massage the dressing into the kale for 2-3 minutes, or until the leaves are dark and softened. Add the Brussels sprouts, quinoa, and cooked asparagus, and toss until combined.
3. Toassemble the bowls, smear a spoonful of hummus along the sideof each bowl. Then portion the kale salad evenly between the four bowls, top

with avocado, egg, and your desired garnishes.
Serve immediately.

To Make the Lemon Vinaigrette:

1. Whisk all ingredients together in a small mixing
   bowl until combined.

5. Green Smoothie With AppleAnd Avocado

Ingredients

2 servings

- 3 cups spinach
- 1 Granny Smith apple, roughly chopped
- 2 cups coconut water
- 1 avocado
- 1 banana, frozen for at least 15 minutes
- 3 tablespoons chia seeds
- 1 teaspoon honey, or more, to taste

Directions

1. Place the spinach, appleand coconut water in a blender, and blend until smooth.

2. Add theavocado, frozen banana, chia seeds and honey, and blend until the mixture is smooth and creamy.

3. Pour the smoothie into tall glasses and serve immediately (while it's still chilled).

6. Avocado Toast with Persimmon, Pomegranateand Fennel

Ingredients

- 1 avocado
- 1 tablespoon goat cheese
- 1/2 tsp. lime juice
- 1/4 tsp. salt
- 2 pieces of bread, toasted
- Thinly sliced persimmon
- Thinly sliced fennel bulb, plus a few fennel fronds
- 2 tablespoons pomegranate seeds
- 2 tsp. honey

Directions

1. Cut theavocado in half. Removeand discard the seed. Scoop the flesh out intoa bowl. Add the goat cheese, lime juiceand salt. Lightly mash with a fork.

2. Spread the mashed avocadoout onto the toast, dividing it evenly between the two slices. Top with a few slices of persimmon and fennel. Then sprinkle with the fennel fronds and pomegranate seeds. Drizzle with honey. Serveand enjoy.

7. Instant Pot Yogurt

Ingredients

- 8 cups whole milk*

- 1/4 cup plain whole milk yogurt

Directions

1. Add milk toa 6-qt Instant Pot; closeand lock the lid. Select yogurt setting; adjust pressure to boil. This can take up to 1 hour.

2. Working carefully, cool the Instant Pot insert in a bowl of ice water, stirring occasionally, until the milk reaches 100 to 110 degrees F, about 15- 20 minutes; set aside 1 cup milk.

3. In a medium bowl, whisk together yogurt and reserved 1 cup milk. Stir into remaining milk, being careful not to scrape the bottom of the insert.

4. Return insert into the Instant Pot. Select yogurt setting, set automatically at 8 hours.

5. Transfer to storage containers; cover and chill until cold, about 6-8 hours, or up to 10 days.

8. Petite Vegetable Frittatas

Ingredients

- 1 red bell pepper diced
- 1 yellow bell pepper diced
- 1 zucchini diced
- 1 small onion diced
- 1 cup Parmesan cheese
- 8 eggs beaten together
- 2 tbsp chives
- salt and pepper to taste
- oliveoil for drizzling

Instructions

1. Preheat oven to 350 degrees. In a large 10 inch skillet heat theoliveoil over medium high heat. Sauté the diced zucchini, onion and red and yellow bell peppers for about 5 minutes until they are slightly soft. Season with salt and pepper. Add the sautéed vegetables to the bottom of a regular sized muffin pan.

2. In another bowl, whisk together 8 eggs and season with salt and pepper and add the chopped chives and parmesan. Fill the remaining area in the muffin tin with theegg, gently stirring the ingredients together. Bake in theoven for 10-12 minutes until theeggs are completely set.

Ingredients

- 1/2 cup Quaker Oats rolled oats

- 1/4 cup chia seeds

- 1 cup milk or water

- pinch of salt and cinnamon

- maple syrup or other sweetener to taste

- 1 cup frozen berries of choice (or yesterday's smoothie leftovers)

- yogurt for topping

- berries for topping

Instructions

1. Place theoats, seeds, milk, salt, and cinnamon in a jar with a lid. Refrigerateovernight.

2. Puree the berries. (I usually incorporate this into my smoothie routine, so I either use leftover smoothieor just blend up a huge smoothie batch so I havea littleextra for theoats. You don't HAVE to do this, but it's a nice way toadd some fruit and color.)

3. Stir oats with your frozen berry pureeand top with yogurt and more berries, nuts, honey, whatevs you like.

Ingredients

4 servings

- 2 tablespoons extra-virgin oliveoil
- 1 onion, minced
- 1 red bell pepper, minced
- 3 garlic cloves, minced
- 2 tablespoons harissa
- One 28-ounce can crushed tomatoes
- 2 teaspoons ground cumin
- 1 teaspoon ground coriander
- Salt and freshly ground black pepper
- 8 largeeggs
- ¼ cup chopped fresh parsley
- ¼ cup chopped fresh cilantro
- Crusty bread, if desired

Directions

1. Preheat theoven to 350°F.

2. In a large, oven-safe skillet, heat theoliveoil over medium heat. Add theonion and bell pepper and sauté until tender, 4 to 5 minutes. Add the garlic and sauté until fragrant, 1 minute more.

3. Stir in the harissaand cook for 1 minute, stirring constantly. Add the tomatoes, stir again and bring toa simmer. Add the cumin and coriander; season with salt and pepper. Simmer 10 to 15 minutes, until the flavor develops.

4. Make 8 wells in the tomato sauceand carefully crack an egg intoeach. Transfer the skillet to theoven and bake until theegg whites are fully set, but the yolks are still slightly jiggly, 23 to 27 minutes.

5. Garnish the shakshuka with parsley and cilantro. Serve immediately with bread for dipping.

11. Baked Smoky Carrot Bacon

Ingredients

- 3 large carrots
- 2 tablespoons rapeseed oil
- 1 teaspoon garlic powder
- 1 teaspoon smoked paprika
- 1 teaspoon salt

Directions

1. Rinse carrot (no need to peel) and slice, lengthwise, using a mandoline. Lay the carrot strips on a baking sheet lined with parchment paper. Preheat oven to 320°F.
2. Stir together remaining ingredients in a small bowl and then brush carrot strips on both sides.
3. Place in theoven for 15 minutes, or when the carrot strips are wavy.

Serves: 4

Cooking Time: 40

Ingredients

For the Pasta:

- 4 cups rigatoni
- 2 tablespoons oliveoil
- 2 tablespoons vegan butter
- 1 medium shallot or red onion, diced
- 1 teaspoon red pepper flakes
- 4 sage leaves, minced
- 2 cups canned pumpkin purée
- 1 1/2 cups almond milk
- A pinch of cinnamon
- A pinch of nutmeg
- 1 bunch of kale, stems removed and leaves coarsely chopped

- 1 cup vegan Parmesan

- Salt and black pepper, to taste

- 2 vegan sausages (optional)

For the Shiitake Bacon:

- 1 8-ounce packageof Shiitake, sliced

- 1 tablespoon tamari

- 1 tablespoon liquid smoke

- 2 tablespoons coconut oil

- 1 tablespoon vegan Worcestershire sauce

- 1 teaspoon red pepper flakes

Directions

To Make the Shiitake Bacon:

1. Slice the mushrooms, coat in all the ingredients and back in theoven on 250°F for 30 minutes. Rotate the mushrooms in between midway for an even cook. Mushrooms should be crispy, not hard.

To Make the Pasta:

1. Bring a large pot of salted water toa boil. Cook the pastaaccording to package directions, until al dente.

2. Meanwhile, in a large skillet, heat theoliveoil and butter over medium heat until the butter is melted. Add the shallots, sage, red pepper flakes, and a pinch of salt. Saute for 3-4 minutes, or until shallots are translucent.

3. Whisk in the pumpkin, cinnamon, nutmeg, and saute for 1 minute, stirring constantly. Stir in thealmond milk and bring toa simmer. Stir in the chopped kaleand simmer for 4-5 minutes, or until slightly thickened. Stir in the vegan Parmesan.

4. Season to taste with salt and black pepper.

5. Toss the pasta with the pumpkin sauceand top with shiitake bacon, vegan Parmesan, and pumpkin seeds.

Serves: 2

Cooking Time: 10

Ingredients

Portobello Mushroom Bacon:

- 1 thinly sliced portobello mushroom (crimini will also work)
- 3 tsp liquid smoke
- 2 tbsp coconut aminos (see notes)
- 1 tbsp maple syrup
- 1 tbsp molasses (or more maple syrup, molasses adds darker notes)
- 1/4 tsp onion powder
- 1/4 tsp salt (or to taste)
- 1/8 tsp chili powder (or 1/4 tsp for more spice)
- 1/8 tsp garlic powder
- 1/8 tsp clove

Whipped Mayo:

- 3 tbsp vegan mayo
- 1 tsp dry mustard powder
- **Toppings:**

- 1 tomato
- 2-4 romaine lettuce leaves
- **Bread:**

- 2 slices of your favorite bread, toasted

Directions

1. Mix all of the ingredients for the portobello mushroom bacon except for the first ingredient (the mushrooms). Stir well and set aside.
2. Lay the sliced mushrooms intoa skillet and pour the bacon flavor mixtureover the bacon.
3. Cook on each side for 3-5 minutes until the mushrooms have cooked down toabout half their original sizeor until the liquid has absorbed and browned on the mushrooms.

4. While the mushrooms are browning, mix your mayoand set aside.

5. Toast your Ezekiel bread (or bread of choice) and spread the mayoon each slice.

6. Thinly slice the tomatoand layer the tomatoand lettuce leaves on the bread. Then, top with bacon.

Serves: 18-24

Ingredients

For the Coconut Bacon:

- 3 cups coconut flakes
- 3 tablespoons soy sauce
- 2 1/2 tablespoons liquid smoke
- 2 tablespoons maple syrup

For the Doughnuts:

- 1 1/4 cup all-purpose flour
- 1/4 teaspoon salt
- 1 teaspoon baking soda
- 1/2 cup almond milk
- 1/3 cup brown sugar
- 1 tablespoon ground flax seed
- 3 tablespoons hot water
- 4 teaspoons coconut oil, melted

- 1 teaspoon vanillaextract

For the Fondant Icing:

- 1 cup of confectioner's sugar or mapleextract
- 1-3 tablespoons of water

Directions

To Make the Coconut Bacon:

1. Combineall the ingredients together in a large bowl distributing evenly and coating well.
2. Layer ontoa sheet pan and bake in a preheated 325°F oven for approximately 10-20 minutes checking throughout baking and tossing to make sure it bakes evenly.

To Make the Doughnuts:

1. Combine ground flax seed with hot water and whisk smooth. Let stand for at least 10 minutes to thicken toa paste.

2. In a large mixing bowl, combine thealmond milk, melted coconut oil, vanillaextract, brown sugar, flax egg, and salt and whisk smooth.

3. Add the sifted flour and baking sodaand whisk smooth.

4. Transfer batter toa pastry bag and pipe half way to the top intoeach of the cavities of a mini or regular sized doughnut mould pan.

5. Bake in a preheated 325°F oven for approximately 8-12 minutes for the minis and about 22 minutes for the larger. When they spring back when gently pressed they are done.

6. Let the doughnuts cool. Then prepare the cube fondant with the mapleextract or 1 cup of confectioners sugar with 1-3 tablespoons water to desired consistency.

7. Dip in icing glazeand then in crispy coconut bacon.

Ingredients

For the Penne:

- 3 medium-sized beets, cleaned and cut intoa small dice
- 3 tablespoons oliveoil, divided
- 3 cloves garlic
- 1/2 cup vegan parmesan cheese, plus more for garnish
- 1/2 cup vegetable stock
- 1/4 cup almond milk
- 1/2 pound gluten-free penne pasta
- Sea salt and freshly ground pepper
- 1/2 cup cashews
- 2 tablespoons nutritional yeast

For the Shiitake Bacon:

- 1 packages of Shiitakes, sliced
- 1 tablespoon tamari

- 1 tablespoon liquid smoke

- 2 tablespoons coconut oil

- 1 tablespoon vegan Worcestershire sauce

- 1 teaspoon red pepper flakes

Directions

To Make the Shiitake Bacon:

1. Slice the mushrooms, coat them with all the ingredients, and bake in theoven at 250°F for 30 minutes.
2. Rotate the mushrooms in midway for an even cook. Mushrooms should be crispy, not hard. (coat in ingredients for however long you can)

To Make the Penne:

1. Preheat oven to 400°F.
2. On a rimmed baking sheet, toss the rinsed and peeled beets in 1 tablespoon. oil.
3. Season them with a good pinch of salt and pepper.
4. Wrap them in aluminum foil.

5. Peel the garlic, and treat it as you did the beets.

6. Roast the vegetables for 40 minutes. Check for doneness at the 30-minute mark.

7. Transfer beets toa food processor.

8. Soak cashews in hot water for a few minutes.

9. Add the roasted garlic, cashews, nutritional yeast, half of the vegan parmesan cheese, and the two remaining tablespoons of oil.

10. Pulse them until they're smooth.

11. Transfer beet mixture toa small saucepan.

12. Add the stock and almond milk and bring it toa light simmer.

13. Add remaining cheeseand another pinch of salt.

14. Simmer it on low for about 2 minutes.

15. Cook the penne until al dente.

16. Drain it and return it toa skillet.

17. Pour the sauceover the pastaand toss it to combine.

18. Top it with additional cheeseand shiitake bacon.

Ingredients

- 1 Portobello mushroom, stump and gills removed, and sliced into 1/8-inch thin slices
- 2 tablespoons tamari
- 2 tablespoons water
- 2-3 teaspoons maple syrup or coconut nectar
- 1/4 teaspoon smoked paprika
- A few pinches of cracked black pepper

Directions

1. Preheat oven to 350°F. Linea baking pan with parchment paper.
2. Place mushroom strips in a shallow dish. Add the marinade ingredients toa jar with a lid and shake to combine. Pour over the sliced mushrooms and tilt the dish to distribute the marinadeover all the strips. Marinate for 15 minutes or up toa few hours if you have time.

3. Place the strip on the prepared pan, leaving a little room between each one. Sprinkleon a littleextrapepper, if desired. Bake for 15 minutes, flip carefully, and continue baking for about 5 more minutes. Remove from oven and let sit on pan while you prepare the sandwiches.

17. Spaghetti With Cauliflower Carbonaraand Tempeh
Bacon

Serves: 2-3

Ingredients

For the Cauliflower Carbonara Sauce:

- 6 cups cauliflower florets (1 medium head)
- 1 cup cooking water
- 1 tablespoon extra virgin oliveoil
- 1/2 cup oat milk, unsweetened (or other non-dairy milk)
- 1/4 cup nutritional yeast
- Mustard, to taste
- Sea salt and black pepper, to taste

For the Bacon:

- 1 packageof smoky tempeh
- Tamari, as needed
- Smoked paprika powder, as needed

For the Spaghetti Carbonara Bowl:

- 4 small zucchini
- Freshly ground black pepper, as needed
- Almond Parmesan, as needed (optional)
- Parsley or chives, as needed (optional)

Directions

To Make the Cauliflower Carbonara Sauce:

1. Cook or steam the cauliflower florets until tender. Don't pour away the cooking liquid, you'll need someof it for the sauce.
2. Put the cauliflower in the blender together with 1 cup of the cooking water, oliveoil, oat milk, nutritional yeast, mustard, salt, and pepper. Blend until smooth.

To Make the Bacon:

1. Cut the smoked tempeh into cubes. Marinate with tamari and smoked paprika to taste.

2. Heat some coconut oil in a frying pan. Bake the tempeh until it's slightly crunchy on theoutside. These will add a deep salty flavor to the pasta.

To Make the Spaghetti Carbonara Bowl:

1. Peel the zucchini if you prefer white pasta instead of green noodles. Cut the zucchini in half and usea spiralizer to turn it into noodles.
2. Mix the zucchini noodles with the warm cauliflower carbonara sauce. Add as much tempeh bacon as your heart desires.
3. Top with freshly ground black pepper, parsley or chives, and almond Parmesan cheese

Serves: 10

Ingredients

For the Potatoes:

- 10 baby Red potatoes
- 3 tablespoons chives, chopped fine
- 3 tablespoons oliveoil

For the Cashew Mozzarella:

- 1/2 cup raw cashews
- 1/4 cup tapioca flour
- 1 1/4 cups water
- 1 1/2 tablespoons nutritional yeast
- 1/2 teaspoon lemon juice
- 1/2 teaspoon white pepper
- 1/2 teaspoon garlic powder
- 3/4 teaspoon sea salt

For the Chipotle Cream:

- 1 cup raw cashews

- 3/4 cup salsa

- 1 teaspoon chili powder

- 1/4 teaspoon sea salt

For the Tempeh Bacon Bits:

- 1 10-ounce packageof tempeh

- 3 tablespoons soy sauceor gluten-free tamari

- 2 tablespoons maple syrup

- 2 teaspoons liquid smoke

- 2 teaspoons red hot sauce

- 1 tablespoon coconut oil

Directions

To Make the Potatoes:

1. Combineall liquid ingredients for the tempeh bacon in a container with a lid, except for the coconut oil.

2. Chop the tempeh into very fine bits and toss it with the marinade. Let sit while the potatoes boil.

3. Bring a pot of water to boil with a sprinkleof salt. Boil the potatoes until fork tender, about 10 minutes.

4. Preheat theoven to 450°F. When the potatoes are cool enough to handle, usea metal spatulaor the bottom of a glass to smash them until they areabout 1/2-3/4 inch thick. Transfer the potatoes toa baking sheet lined with foil and a small amount of oil. Drizzle the potatoes with 3 tablespoons oliveoil and bake for 20 minutes.

5. While the potatoes are baking, prepare the cashew mozzarella, chipotle cream, and finish preparing the tempeh bacon bits.

To Make the Cashew Mozzarella:

1. Soak the cashews for two hours or overnight to soften. I recommend keeping soaked and drained cashews on hand in your freezer to speed things along. You can also boil them for ten minutes to saveon time.

2. In a high powered blender, add the soaked cashews and remaining mozzarella ingredients. Blend on high for two minutes until mixture is smooth.

3. Transfer toa saucepan on medium high heat and stir until the cheese forms a gooey ball in the center, about 5 minutes.

To Make the Tempeh Bacon Bits:

1. After 10-15 minutes of marinating the tempeh bits, melt the coconut oil in skillet over medium heat. Add the marinated tempeh bacon bits to the skillet and cook for 10-12 minutes, stirring often to prevent sticking. You want the tempeh bacon bits to bea bit blackened and sticky. You may have toadd a bit moreoil or water to deglaze the pan as you go.

To Make the Chipotle Cream:

1. Soak the cashews for two hours or overnight, then drain. Add the soaked cashews toa blender with remaining ingredients and blend on high for 2-3 minutes until smooth.

ToAssemble:

1. Remove the potatoes from theoven and top each one with a spoonful of cashew mozzarella. Bake for

another 5 minutes until cheese becomes melty. Finish each Vegan Loaded Smashed Potato with a large dollop of chipotle cream, tempeh bacon bits, and chives.

Serves: 8

Ingredients

For the Tofu Bacon:

- 1 14-ounce block of extra firm tofu
- Oil of choice (optional)
- 2/3 cup water
- 1/3 cup soy sauce
- 1/4 cup brown sugar or maple syrup (optional)
- 1 tablespoon vegan Worcestershire sauce
- 1 tablespoon liquid smoke
- 1 tablespoon smoked paprika (optional)

For the Bagel:

- 3 1/2 cups all-purpose flour
- 1 1/4 cups warm water
- 2 teaspoons active dry yeast
- 1 1/2 tablespoons white sugar
- 1 1/2 teaspoons salt

- 1 teaspoon sesame seeds

- 1 teaspoon poppy seeds

- 1/2 teaspoon black sesame seeds

- 1/2 teaspoon onion flakes

- 1/2 teaspoon coarse salt

- 3 liters of water

- 1 teaspoon salt

- 1 teaspoon baking soda

For the Topping:

- Vegan mayonnaise

- Romaine lettuce

- Tomato

Directions

To Make the Tofu Bacon:

1. Mix together the water, soy sauce, maple syrup or brown sugar, vegan Worcestershire sauce, liquid smoke, and smoked paprika (if using). Place the

marinade in a rectangular container that fits the block of tofu.

2. If you have the time, press your tofu in between two paper towels (or in a tofu press) to get someof the liquid out, then slice into thin and even slices.

3. Place the tofu in the marinadeand place in the refrigerator for 24-48 hours.

4. Place the tofu strips on a non-stick silicone baking mat or parchment paper and bake for 1 1/2 to 2 hours at 200°F. Alternatively, you can do this in a food dehydrator. Keep flipping the tofu every 30 minutes.

5. While you're baking the tofu, you can start to make the bagels.

To Make the Bagels:

1. Place the water, sugar, and yeast in a small bowl and let the yeast activate for 10 minutes.

2. In a large mixing bowl, mix the flour and salt together. Once the yeast has activated, mix the water mixture into the dry ingredients and mix well. Knead for 5-7 minutes until the dough is smooth and elastic. Let rise for 1 hour while covered with a kitchen towel.

3. Mix all of your bagel toppings (sesame seeds, poppy seeds, coarse salt, and onion flakes) in a small bowl.

4. Boil 3 liters of water with the 1 teaspoon of salt and baking soda. Once boiling, lower the heat and shape your bagels once the hour has elapsed.

5. Takeout your dough and divide it intoeight equal pieces. To form the bagels, form each piece intoa small bun and lay them on a hard surface. While keeping the seams (if any) underneath, from the top, poke the middleof the bun with oneof your index fingers. Once your index has reached the hard surface beneath, pick up the bagel and enlarge the hole so that your two index fingers by making a circular motion.

6. Placeon the baking mat until you have shaped all of the bagels.

7. Place the bagels into the boiling water for 45 seconds to 1 minuteon each side.

8. Once the time has elapsed, place the bagels on the baking sheet and top with the seeds.

9. Bake for 25 minutes, start checking them at the 25-minute mark. Bake longer if needed. Placeon a cooling rack.

10. Fry your tofu bacon in a frying pan with a bit of cooking spay or oil of choice. Fry on both sides as desired.

11. Toassemble, layer your bagel with some vegan mayonnaise, a sliceof tomato, some tofu bacon strips, and some salt and pepper.

Serves: 8-10

Cooking Time: 30

Ingredients

For the TVP Chili:

- 1 cup textured vegetable protein (TVP)
- 1 cup water, divided
- 1 vegan beef-flavored bouillon cube
- 1 15-ounce can crushed tomatoes
- 2 teaspoons chili powder
- 1 teaspoon taco seasoning (optional)
- 1/2 teaspoon cumin
- 1/2 teaspoon cayenne powder
- Salt and pepper, to taste

For the TVP Bacon:

- 2 tablespoons vegetableoil
- 1/2 cup textured vegetable protein (TVP)

- 1/4 cup, plus 2 tablespoons boiling water

- 1/2 vegan chicken bouillon cube

- 1/2 teaspoon liquid smoke

- 1/4 teaspoon veganWorcestershire sauce

For the Beer Cheese Sauce:

- 1/2 cup favorite lager or golden ale

- 1 cup vegan cheddar shreds

- 1 cup vegan pepperjack shreds

For the Tater Tot Nachos:

- Beer cheese sauce (recipeabove)

- TVP bacon (recipeabove)

- 1 extra largeor family-size bag of tater tots (or 3 small bags)

- Guacamole (homemadeor store bought)

- Vegan sour cream

- Pico de gallo (homemadeor store bought)

- Jalapeños

- Cilantro

- Green onion

- Black olives
- Any other garnishes you likeon your nachos

Directions

To Prep:

1. Preheat oven and cook tater tots according to package directions.

To Make the TVP Chili:

1. In a bowl, add dry TVP. Heat 3/4 cup water and vegan beef bouillon until boiling, then add boiling water to TVP, mixing to combine. Set aside to rehydrate for 10 minutes.
2. Add rehydrated TVP, crushed tomatoes, remaining 1/4 water, and seasoning toa small pot. Bring toa boil, cover and simmer on low, stirring every 10 minutes or so.

To Make the TVP Bacon:

1. While your chili is simmering, make your TVP bacon In a bowl, add dry TVP.

2. Heat water and vegan chicken bouillon until boiling, then add boiling water to TVP, mixing to combine. Set aside to rehydrate for 10 minutes. Add seasonings and mix again to combine.

3. In a small pan, heat oil on medium-high heat. Add TVP and stir constantly until the TVP becomes darker in color and crispy, much resembling real bacon bits, about 10-15 minutes.

4. Transfer TVP bacon bits toa paper towel-lined plateand set aside until ready to be used.

To Make the Beer Cheese Sauce:

1. In a saucepan on medium heat, add both cheeses. Stir constantly until the cheese starts to melt a little.

2. Add beer slowly (1/4 cup at a time) and continue to stir the cheese sauce until it is freeof clumps.

3. Bring toa slow boil, stirring constantly so you let someof the beer cook out.

4. Turn heat to low, and simmer for about 15 minutes, stirring often.

5. Once cheese sauce is done, you can start to assemble your tater tot nachos.

ToAssemble:

1. In a deep skillet or baking dish, lay half the chili on the bottom.
2. Add half of the tater tots, then cheese sauce, then the rest of the chili. Add the remaining tater tots, chili, and nacho cheese.
3. Garnish with TVP bacon, guacamole, cilantro, jalapeños, green onion, pico de gallo, and any other topping you loveon your nachos.

21. Banana Bread

Prep time: 10 minutes

Cook time: 55 minutes

Yield: Makes one loaf

Ingredients

- 2 to 3 very ripe bananas, peeled (about 1 1/4 to 1 1/2 cups mashed)
- 1/3 cup melted butter, unsalted or salted
- 1 teaspoon baking soda
- Pinch of salt
- 3/4 cup sugar (1/2 cup if you would like it less sweet, 1 cup if more sweet)
- 1 largeegg, beaten
- 1 teaspoon vanillaextract
- 1 1/2 cups of all-purpose flour

Directions

1. Preheat theoven to 350°F (175°C), and butter a 4x8-inch loaf pan.

2. In a mixing bowl, mash the ripe bananas with a fork until completely smooth. Stir the melted butter into the mashed bananas.

3. Mix in the baking sodaand salt. Stir in the sugar, beaten egg, and vanillaextract. Mix in the flour.

4. Pour the batter into your prepared loaf pan. Bake for 50 minutes to 1 hour at 350°F (175°C), or until a tester inserted into the center comes out clean.

5. Remove from oven and let cool in the pan for a few minutes. Then remove the banana bread from the pan and let cool completely before serving. Sliceand serve. (A bread knife helps to make slices that aren't crumbly.)

Prep Time: 5 Mins

Total Time: 20 Mins

Yields: 12

Ingredients

- 12 largeeggs
- water

Directions

1. Placeeggs in a large pot and cover by an inch of cold water. Place pot on stoveand bring toa boil. Instantly turn off heat and cover pot. Let sit for 11 minutes.
2. Remove from pan and transfer ice water. Let cool 2 minutes before peeling and serving.

Prep Time: 10 Min

Cook Time: 40 Min

Total Time: 50 Min

Serve: 5

Ingredients

- Fresh vegetables
- 2 teaspoons oil
- Breast milk or formula
- Some suggestions for vegetables to roast include:
- Potato
- Kumara
- Yam
- Carrot
- Parsnip
- Pumpkin

Directions

1. Preheat theoven to 180 degrees Celsius.
2. Peel and slice vegetables.
3. Drizzle with oil.

4. Place in an oven tray and bake for 30 to 40 minutes until soft.

5. Remove from theoven and leave to cool for five minutes.

6. Mash with a potato masher. Or purée in a food processor or blender until smooth.

7. Stir through enough breast milk or formula to makea smooth purée.

8. Freeze leftover cooled purée in ice cube trays.

24. Butternut Squash Rossoto

Prep Time: 15 Mins

Total Time: 55 Mins

Yields: 8 Servings

Ingredients

- 7 c. low-sodium chicken broth
- 1 tbsp. extra-virgin oliveoil
- 1 small onion, chopped
- 2 tbsp. butter, divided
- 4 c. cubed butternut squash (from a 2 1/2-lb. squash)
- 3 cloves garlic, minced
- 2 c. arborio rice
- 1/2 c. white wine
- 1 c. freshly grated Parmesan
- 2 tbsp. freshly chopped sage

Directions

1. In a medium saucepan over medium heat, bring chicken broth toa simmer. Reduce heat to low.
2. In a large pot or Dutch oven, heat oil. Add onion and cook, stirring often, until beginning to soften, about 5

minutes. Stir in squash, 1 tablespoon butter and garlic. Cook until the squash is beginning to color around edges and then soft, about 6 minutes. Season with salt and pepper.

3. Stir in remaining tablespoon butter arborio rice, stirring quickly. Cook until the grains are well-coated and smell slightly toasty, about 2 minutes. Add the wineand cook until the wine has mostly absorbed.

4. With a ladle, add about 1 cup hot broth. Stirring often, cook until the rice has mostly absorbed liquid. Add remaining broth about 1 cup at a time, continuing toallow the rice toabsorb each addition of broth beforeadding more.

5. Stir often and cook until squash is tender and risotto is al denteand creamy, not mushy, about 25 minutes. Stir in Parmesan and sage, then season with salt and pepper before serving.

Total: 55 min

Prep: 10 min

Cook: 45 min

Yield: 10 to 12 servings

Ingredients

- 4 large sweet potatoes, scrubbed
- Kosher salt and freshly ground black pepper
- 2 cups heavy cream
- 2 bay leaves
- 1/2 teaspoon ground cinnamon
- Pinch freshly grated nutmeg
- 1/2 orange, zested
- 2 tablespoons brown sugar
- 1 tablespoon unsalted butter

Directions

1. Preheat theoven to 350 degrees F.

2. Prick the sweet potatoes all over with a fork, drizzle with oliveoil and season with salt and pepper. Put them in a roasting pan and roast for 45 minutes until they are very soft. Remove the pan from theoven.

3. In a small sauce pot, over low heat, heat the cream with the bay leaves, then keep warm until ready to puree potatoes. Discard the bay leaves beforeadding to potatoes.

4. When the potatoes are cool enough to handle, scoop the flesh into the bowl of a food processor. Season with salt, cinnamon, nutmeg, orange zest, and brown sugar. Add cream and 1 tablespoon of butter and puree until super smooth.

Preparation Time: Less Than 30 Mins

Cooking Time: 10 To 30 Mins

Serves: Serves 3–4

Ingredients

- 1 tbsp oliveoil
- 1 onion, roughly chopped
- 2 large carrots, peeled and roughly chopped
- 4cm/1½ inches fresh root ginger, finely chopped
- 1 garlic clove, crushed
- ½ tsp dried red chilli flakes
- 700g/1lb 10oz sweet potatoes, peeled and cubed
- 1.2 litres/2 pints vegetable stock
- salt and freshly ground black pepper

Directions

1. Heat theoil in a large, lidded saucepan over a medium-high heat. Add theonion and carrots and cook until softened. Stir in the ginger, garlic and chilli flakes and fry for 2–3 minutes, or until fragrant.

2. Stir in the sweet potatoes and stock. Turn up the heat and bring the pan to the boil. Reduce the heat to low and simmer with the lid on for 15 minutes, or until the sweet potato is tender.

3. Remove the pan from the heat and blend the soup, using a stick blender, until smooth. Alternatively, tip it intoa food processor and blend. Season to tasteand serve.

27. Blueberry Soup

Prep Time: 5 Min

Cooking Time: 15 Min

Total Time: 20 Min

Serve: 2 to 3

Ingredients

- 3 cups blueberries, fresh or frozen
- 2 tablespoons honey
- 2 teaspoons lemon juice
- 1 cinnamon stick, optional
- 2 teaspoons cornstarch
- 1 teaspoon lemon zest
- Yogurt for serving, if desired

Directions

1. Combine the berries with the honey, lemon juice, cinnamon stick if using (it's traditional, but I generally don't useany) and a cup of water. Bring toa gentle boil, then turn down toa low simmer, cover and cook 8-10 minutes, until the berries are stewed. (At this point, it's also traditional to strain

the berry skins out and just use the juice, but I like to leave them in for more texture.)

2. Stir the cornstarch into 1 Tbs. of warm water to makea slurry, then stir this into the cooked berries. Bring back toa very gentle boil and cook, stirring, until starting to thicken, about 2 minutes. Remove from the heat and stir in the lemon zest.

3. Serve warm, or chill and serve later. Top with a scoop of yogurt before serving (or use whipped cream or creme fraiche instead of yogurt if you'd like to make this a dessert).

Total: 50 mins

Servings: 8

Ingredients

- 1 tablespoon butter
- 1 tablespoon extra-virgin oliveoil
- 1 medium onion, chopped
- 1 stalk celery, chopped
- 2 cloves garlic, chopped
- 1 teaspoon chopped fresh thymeor parsley
- 5 cups chopped carrots
- 2 cups water
- 4 cups reduced-sodium chicken broth, "no-chicken" broth (see Note) or vegetable broth
- ½ cup half-and-half (optional)
- ½ teaspoon salt
- Freshly ground pepper to taste

Directions

Step 1

Heat butter and oil in a Dutch oven over medium heat until the butter melts. Add onion and celery; cook, stirring occasionally, until softened, 4 to 6 minutes. Add garlic and thyme (or parsley); cook, stirring, until fragrant, about 10 seconds.

Step 2

Stir in carrots. Add water and broth; bring toa lively simmer over high heat. Reduce heat to maintain a lively simmer and cook until very tender, about 25 minutes.

Step 3

Puree the soup in batches in a blender until smooth. (Use caution when pureeing hot liquids.) Stir in half-and-half (if using), salt and pepper.

Prep Time: 1 Hour 10 Mins

Total Time: 2 Hours

Yield: Makes 8 cups

Direction

Step 1

Melt butter in a large Dutch oven over low heat. Add onions and next 2 ingredients, and cook, stirring often, 30 to 35 minutes or until onions are caramel colored. (Adjust heat to prevent scorching.) Add apples, and cook, stirring often, 5 minutes. Add broth and next 2 ingredients. Increase heat to medium, and bring toa boil, stirring occasionally. Reduce heat to medium-low, and simmer, stirring occasionally, 20 to 25 minutes or until apples and potatoare tender. Remove from heat, and let stand 15 minutes. Discard bay leaf.

Step 2

Process mixture with a handheld blender until smooth. Add cream and lemon juice. Return to low heat; simmer, stirring often, 15 minutes. Add salt and pepper. Serve with Cheese Puff Pastries.

Prep: 10 Min

Cook: 30 Min

Total Time: 40 Min

Makes: 12 servings (3 quarts)

Ingredients

- 3 cans (14-1/2 ounces each) chicken broth
- 2 cans (15-1/4 ounces each) lima beans, rinsed and drained
- 3 medium carrots, thinly sliced
- 2 medium potatoes, peeled and diced
- 2 small sweet red peppers, chopped
- 2 small onions, chopped
- 2 celery ribs, thinly sliced
- 1/4 cup butter
- 1-1/2 teaspoons dried marjoram
- 1/2 teaspoon salt
- 1/2 teaspoon pepper

- 1/2 teaspoon dried oregano
- 1 cup half-and-half cream
- 3 bacon strips, cooked and crumbled

Directions

1. In a Dutch oven or soup kettle, combine the first 12 ingredients; bring toa boil over medium heat. Reduce heat; cover and simmer for 25-35 minutes or until vegetables are tender.
2. Add cream; heat through but do not boil. Sprinkle with bacon just before serving.